How to Eat for Gastroparesis

Guides, Tips and Recipes To Manage Digestive Health.

Michael Samuel

TABLE OF CONTENTS

Introduction

Living with gastroparesis can be challenging, but understanding the condition and learning how to manage it can significantly improve your quality of life. This book aims to provide comprehensive guides, practical tips, and delicious recipes to help you navigate your journey with gastroparesis. Whether you have just been diagnosed or have been living with the condition for years, the information and strategies outlined in this book will empower you to take control of your digestive health.

Gastroparesis is a chronic condition where the stomach's ability to empty its contents is delayed, causing various digestive symptoms. While there is no cure for gastroparesis, lifestyle modifications, dietary adjustments, and medical treatments can help manage the symptoms and improve overall well-being. This book covers all aspects of living with gastroparesis, from understanding the condition to meal planning and emotional well-being. Let's embark on this journey together to better manage gastroparesis and enhance your digestive health.

1. Understanding Gastroparesis

What is Gastroparesis?

Gastroparesis is a condition characterized by delayed gastric emptying, where the stomach takes longer than normal to empty its contents into the small intestine. This delay can lead to various symptoms, such as nausea, vomiting, bloating, and early satiety (feeling full quickly). The term "gastroparesis" literally means "stomach paralysis," which reflects the reduced motility (movement) of the stomach muscles. In a healthy digestive system, coordinated muscle contractions help move food through the digestive tract. However, in gastroparesis, these contractions are weakened or disrupted, leading to delayed gastric emptying.

Causes and Risk Factors

The exact cause of gastroparesis is often unknown, but several factors can contribute to the development of this condition:

1. **Diabetes:** Diabetes, particularly poorly controlled blood sugar levels, is one of the most common causes of gastroparesis. High blood sugar levels can damage the vagus nerve, which controls stomach muscles, leading to delayed gastric emptying.

2. **Surgery:** Certain surgical procedures, especially those involving the stomach or esophagus, can damage the vagus nerve or other nerves controlling stomach motility, resulting in gastroparesis.

3. **Viral Infections:** Viral infections affecting the stomach can cause temporary or permanent damage to the nerves and muscles, leading to gastroparesis.

4. **Medications:** Some medications, such as narcotics and certain antidepressants, can slow gastric emptying and contribute to gastroparesis.

5. **Autoimmune Diseases:** Autoimmune conditions, where the body's immune system mistakenly attacks its own tissues, can also affect the nerves and muscles of the stomach.

6. **Idiopathic:** In many cases, the cause of gastroparesis is unknown (idiopathic). Researchers continue to study potential genetic, environmental, and other factors that may contribute to the condition.

Symptoms and Diagnosis

Gastroparesis can present with a range of symptoms, which can vary in severity from person to person. Common symptoms include:

- Nausea and vomiting
- Bloating and abdominal distension
- Early satiety (feeling full quickly)

- Weight loss or malnutrition
- Abdominal pain or discomfort
- Acid reflux or heartburn

If you experience these symptoms, it is essential to seek medical evaluation for an accurate diagnosis. Diagnosing gastroparesis typically involves several steps:

1. **Medical History and Physical Examination:** Your doctor will take a detailed medical history and perform a physical examination to assess your symptoms and overall health.

2. **Gastric Emptying Study:** This test measures how quickly food leaves your stomach. It involves eating a small, radioactive-labeled meal, and then a scanner tracks the movement of the meal through your digestive system.

3. **Endoscopy:** An endoscopy allows the doctor to visually examine the inside of your stomach and rule out other potential causes of your symptoms, such as blockages or ulcers.

4. **Other Tests:** Additional tests, such as a barium X-ray, breath test, or gastric manometry (measuring stomach muscle contractions), may be used to further evaluate gastric emptying and motility.

Living with Gastroparesis

Managing gastroparesis involves a combination of dietary changes, lifestyle modifications, and medical treatments. While it may take time to find the right balance, many people with gastroparesis can lead fulfilling lives by making informed choices about their health.

1. **Dietary Changes:** Following a gastroparesis-friendly diet is crucial. This typically involves eating smaller, more frequent meals, avoiding high-fat and high-fiber foods, and opting for easily digestible options. Pureed or liquid meals can also be beneficial.

2. **Lifestyle Modifications:** Simple changes, such as chewing food thoroughly, sitting upright during and after meals, and staying hydrated, can help improve digestion and reduce symptoms.

3. **Medications:** Medications that stimulate stomach motility or help manage symptoms like nausea and vomiting may be prescribed by your doctor. It's essential to follow your doctor's recommendations and discuss any side effects or concerns.

4. **Emotional Well-being:** Living with a chronic condition can be emotionally challenging. Seeking support from friends, family, or support groups, and practicing stress-reduction techniques like mindfulness and relaxation exercises, can positively impact your mental health.

By understanding gastroparesis and implementing the strategies outlined in this book, you can take proactive steps to manage your symptoms and improve your quality of life.

The following chapters will delve deeper into these topics, providing practical guides, tips, and delicious recipes tailored to your needs.

Part I:

Guides to Managing Gastroparesis

2. Dietary Guidelines

Diet plays a crucial role in managing gastroparesis. By making thoughtful choices about what and how you eat, you can help alleviate symptoms and improve your overall quality of life. This chapter provides essential dietary guidelines to help you navigate your food choices and meal planning effectively.

Importance of Diet in Gastroparesis Management

Dietary management is fundamental in controlling the symptoms of gastroparesis. Since the stomach's ability to empty its contents is impaired, the type, consistency, and quantity of food consumed can significantly impact how well the digestive system functions. A well-planned diet can help:

- - Reduce symptoms such as nausea, vomiting, bloating, and abdominal pain.
- - Ensure adequate nutrition and prevent malnutrition.
- - Maintain a healthy weight.
- - Improve overall well-being and quality of life.

Foods to Eat and Avoid

Understanding which foods are easier on your digestive system and which ones to avoid is key to managing gastroparesis.

Foods to Eat:

1. **Low-Fat Foods:** Fat slows gastric emptying, so choose low-fat options. For example, lean

meats, skinless poultry, fish, low-fat dairy products, and egg whites.

2. **Low-Fiber Foods:** High-fiber foods can be difficult to digest and may exacerbate symptoms. Opt for refined grains like white bread, white rice, and low-fiber cereals.

3. **Soft, Well-Cooked Vegetables:** Cook vegetables until they are soft to make them easier to digest. Peeling vegetables can also reduce fiber content.

4. **Fruits Without Skins or Seeds:** Choose canned or cooked fruits, and avoid raw fruits with tough skins or seeds.

5. **Pureed or Liquid Foods:** Soups, smoothies, and pureed meals can be easier to digest and help ensure adequate nutrient intake.

6. **Small, Frequent Meals:** Eating smaller, more frequent meals can prevent the stomach from becoming too full and help manage symptoms.

Foods to Avoid:

1. **High-Fat Foods:** Avoid fried foods, fatty meats, full-fat dairy products, and heavy sauces.

2. **High-Fiber Foods:** Steer clear of whole grains, raw vegetables, legumes, nuts, and seeds.
3. **Carbonated Beverages:** These can cause bloating and discomfort.
4. **Hard-to-Digest Foods:** Foods with skins, seeds, and tough textures, like corn, peas, and berries, should be avoided.
5. **Spicy and Acidic Foods:** These can irritate the stomach lining and worsen symptoms.

Nutritional Considerations

Maintaining proper nutrition is vital for individuals with gastroparesis. Due to the limitations imposed by the condition, it is essential to focus on nutrient-dense foods that provide adequate calories, vitamins, and minerals.

1. **Protein:** Ensure sufficient protein intake to maintain muscle mass and overall health. Lean meats, poultry, fish, eggs, and dairy products are good sources.

2. **Carbohydrates:** Opt for easily digestible carbohydrates like white bread, rice, pasta, and low-fiber cereals. These can provide necessary energy without straining the digestive system.

3. **Fats:** While high-fat foods should be limited, some healthy fats are essential. Small amounts of healthy fats from sources like avocados, olive oil, and nut butters (if tolerated) can be included.

4. **Vitamins and Minerals:** Gastroparesis can lead to deficiencies in vitamins and minerals. Consider taking a multivitamin supplement and focus on nutrient-rich foods. Work with a healthcare provider to monitor and address any deficiencies.

5. **Hydration:** Staying hydrated is crucial. Sip on water throughout the day and include hydrating foods like soups and smoothies. Avoid large amounts of liquid with meals to prevent fullness.

Role of Fiber in the Diet

Fiber plays a complex role in the diet of someone with gastroparesis. While dietary fiber is generally beneficial for digestive health, it can be problematic for those with delayed gastric emptying. High-fiber foods can be difficult to digest and may worsen symptoms. However, not all fiber needs to be eliminated from the diet.

Types of Fiber:

1. **Soluble Fiber:** This type of fiber dissolves in water and forms a gel-like substance. It can be easier to digest and may be better tolerated in small amounts. Sources include oats, peeled apples, and bananas.
2. **Insoluble Fiber:** This type of fiber does not dissolve in water and can add bulk to the stool, which may be harder for the stomach to process. Sources include whole grains, nuts, and raw vegetables.

Managing Fiber Intake:

- - Gradual Introduction: Introduce small amounts of soluble fiber slowly and monitor tolerance.

- - Cooking and Pureeing: Cooking vegetables and fruits can break down fiber and make them easier to digest. Pureeing foods can further reduce fiber content.
- - Monitoring Symptoms: Keep a food diary to track fiber intake and its impact on symptoms. Adjust your diet based on your body's responses.

By following these dietary guidelines and making informed food choices, you can better manage gastroparesis symptoms and maintain optimal nutritional health. The next chapter will delve into practical tips for meal planning and preparation, helping you create a balanced and manageable eating routine.

3. Meal Planning and Preparation

Managing gastroparesis requires thoughtful meal planning and preparation. The right strategies can help you enjoy a variety of foods while minimizing symptoms. This chapter provides practical tips and guidelines for effective meal planning, creating balanced meal plans, preparing food safely, and making smart shopping choices for gastroparesis-friendly foods.

Tips for Effective Meal Planning

Effective meal planning is essential for managing gastroparesis. By planning your meals in advance, you can ensure that you have suitable food options readily available, reduce stress, and prevent symptom flare-ups.

1. **Plan Small, Frequent Meals:** Aim for six to eight small meals a day instead of three large ones. This can prevent your stomach from becoming too full and help manage symptoms.

2. **Choose Easily Digestible Foods:** Focus on low-fat, low-fiber, and soft or pureed foods that are easier for your stomach to process.

3. Incorporate Nutrient-Dense Options:
Ensure that each meal contains a balance of protein, carbohydrates, and healthy fats. This helps maintain energy levels and nutritional status.

4. Stay Hydrated: Include hydrating foods and beverages, but avoid drinking large amounts of liquids with meals to prevent fullness and discomfort.

5. Prepare Meals in Advance: Cook and store meals in portion-sized containers to save time and make it easier to eat small, frequent meals throughout the day.

Creating a Balanced Meal Plan

A balanced meal plan ensures that you receive adequate nutrition while managing gastroparesis symptoms. Here's a step-by-step guide to creating a meal plan that works for you:

1. **Identify Safe Foods:** Make a list of foods that you tolerate well. Include a variety of proteins, carbohydrates, and fats to ensure nutritional balance.

2. **Set a Schedule:** Plan to eat every 2-3 hours. This keeps your stomach from getting too full and helps maintain stable energy levels.

3. **Mix and Match:** Create meals that combine protein, carbohydrates, and fats. For example, a small meal might include a portion of lean chicken, mashed potatoes, and a small serving of steamed carrots.

4. **Use Soft and Pureed Foods:** Incorporate soups, smoothies, and pureed dishes into your meal plan. These can be easier to digest and provide essential nutrients.

5. **Monitor Portion Sizes:** Keep portions small to avoid overloading your stomach. Use measuring cups or a food scale to ensure consistency.

6. **Include Snacks:** Plan for nutritious snacks between meals. Options like yogurt, applesauce, or a small smoothie can keep you satisfied without overwhelming your stomach.

Preparing and Cooking Food Safely

Safe food preparation and cooking techniques are vital for individuals with gastroparesis. Proper methods can make food easier to digest and reduce the risk of gastrointestinal distress.

1. **Cook Thoroughly:** Ensure that all foods are cooked thoroughly to make them easier to digest. Use methods like baking, steaming, boiling, or slow cooking.

2. **Avoid High-Fat Cooking Methods:** Steer clear of frying or using excessive oil, as high-fat foods can delay gastric emptying and worsen symptoms.

3. **Puree and Blend:** Pureeing or blending foods can reduce their texture and make them easier to swallow and digest. Soups, smoothies, and pureed vegetables are excellent options.

4. **Chew Food Well:** Encourage thorough chewing to break down food into smaller, more manageable pieces. This aids digestion and reduces the workload on your stomach.

5. **Avoid High-Fiber Additions:** Limit the use of high-fiber ingredients like whole grains, raw vegetables, and legumes. Instead, focus on low-fiber, easily digestible options.

Smart Shopping Tips for Gastroparesis-Friendly Foods

Smart shopping can help you stock your kitchen with foods that support your dietary needs and reduce the likelihood of symptom flare-ups.

1. **Create a Shopping List:** Make a list of gastroparesis-friendly foods before heading to

the store. This ensures you buy what you need and avoid impulse purchases.

2. **Focus on Low-Fat and Low-Fiber Options:** Choose lean proteins, low-fat dairy products, and refined grains. Avoid high-fat and high-fiber items that can be harder to digest.

3. **Opt for Soft and Pureed Foods:** Look for canned or cooked fruits without skins or seeds, soft-cooked vegetables, and prepared soups. These can be easier to digest and convenient.

4. **Check Labels:** Read food labels to avoid high-fat, high-fiber, and highly processed foods. Look for simple, whole-food ingredients that are easier on your digestive system.

5. **Buy in Bulk:** Purchase staple items like rice, pasta, and low-fiber cereals in bulk. This ensures you always have gastroparesis-friendly options on hand.

6. **Consider Frozen Options:** Frozen fruits and vegetables can be a convenient and nutritious choice. They are often picked at peak ripeness and can be easily cooked or blended.

By implementing these meal planning and preparation strategies, you can effectively manage your gastroparesis symptoms and maintain a balanced, nutritious diet. The next chapter will provide detailed recipes tailored to the dietary needs of individuals with gastroparesis, offering delicious and easy-to-digest meal options.

4. Eating Habits and Lifestyle Changes

Successfully managing gastroparesis involves more than just what you eat—how you eat and your daily habits can significantly impact your symptoms. This chapter focuses on essential eating habits and lifestyle changes that can help you manage gastroparesis more effectively.

Eating Small, Frequent Meals

One of the most important strategies for managing gastroparesis is to eat small, frequent meals throughout the day. This approach helps prevent your stomach from becoming too full, which can exacerbate symptoms like nausea and bloating.

Benefits of Small, Frequent Meals:

1. **Easier Digestion:** Smaller meals are less taxing on your stomach and can move more efficiently through your digestive system.
2. **Stable Blood Sugar Levels:** Eating more frequently can help maintain stable blood sugar levels, which is particularly beneficial for individuals with diabetes.
3. **Reduced Symptoms:** Smaller meals are less likely to trigger symptoms such as nausea, vomiting, and bloating.

Tips for Implementing Small, Frequent Meals:

- **Meal Timing:** Aim to eat every 2-3 hours. Set reminders if necessary to ensure you don't skip meals.
- **Portion Control:** Use smaller plates and bowls to help control portion sizes. Measure portions to maintain consistency.
- **Balanced Nutrition:** Ensure each meal includes a balance of protein, carbohydrates, and healthy fats to provide sustained energy.

Proper Chewing and Food Texture

How you chew your food and the texture of the food you eat can significantly affect your digestion. Proper chewing and choosing the right food textures can help ease the digestive process.

Importance of Proper Chewing:

- **Breaks Down Food:** Chewing thoroughly breaks food into smaller pieces, making it easier for your stomach to process.
- **Mixes with Saliva:** Chewing mixes food with saliva, which contains enzymes that begin the digestive process.

Tips for Proper Chewing:

- - **Chew Slowly:** Take your time with each bite, chewing thoroughly until the food is a smooth consistency.
- - **Mindful Eating:** Focus on your meal without distractions. This helps you chew more thoroughly and enjoy your food.

Food Texture Considerations:

- - **Soft Foods:** Soft and well-cooked foods are generally easier to digest. Examples include mashed potatoes, scrambled eggs, and tender cooked vegetables.
- - **Pureed Foods:** Pureeing foods can help reduce their texture, making them easier

to swallow and digest. Soups, smoothies, and pureed fruits and vegetables are good options.
- **- Avoid Hard and Crunchy Foods:** These can be difficult to chew and digest, potentially worsening symptoms.

Staying Hydrated

Staying hydrated is crucial for overall health, but it is particularly important for individuals with gastroparesis. Proper hydration can help maintain digestive health and prevent complications.

Benefits of Hydration:

- Aids Digestion: Adequate fluid intake helps move food through the digestive tract and prevent constipation.
- Prevents Dehydration: Frequent vomiting, a common symptom of gastroparesis, can lead to dehydration, making it essential to replenish lost fluids.

Tips for Staying Hydrated:

- **- Sip Fluids Throughout the Day:** Drink small amounts of fluids consistently rather than consuming large quantities at once, which can cause fullness.
- **- Choose Hydrating Foods:** Foods with high water content, such as soups, broths, and fruits like watermelon and cucumbers, can contribute to your fluid intake.
- **- Avoid High-Sugar Beverages:** Sugary drinks can cause bloating and discomfort. Opt for water, herbal teas, and clear broths instead.
- **- Monitor Your Intake:** Aim for at least 8-10 cups of fluid daily, adjusting based on your specific needs and activity level.

Lifestyle Changes to Improve Digestion

In addition to dietary adjustments, certain lifestyle changes can enhance your digestive health and help manage gastroparesis symptoms.

Physical Activity:

- **Light Exercise:** Gentle activities like walking can stimulate digestion and help food move through your digestive tract. Aim for a short walk after meals to aid digestion.
- **Avoid Strenuous Exercise:** Intense physical activity can worsen symptoms. Stick to low-impact exercises that don't strain your stomach.

Stress Management:

- **Reduce Stress:** Stress can exacerbate gastroparesis symptoms. Engage in stress-reducing activities such as yoga, meditation, or deep breathing exercises.
- Adequate Rest: Ensure you get enough sleep and rest. Fatigue can worsen digestive issues and overall well-being.

Eating Environment:

- Sit Upright During and After Meals: Eating while sitting upright can help gravity assist in the digestive process. Avoid lying down for at least 1-2 hours after eating.

- Create a Relaxing Atmosphere: Eat in a calm, pleasant environment without distractions. This can promote better digestion and mindful eating.

Avoiding Smoking and Alcohol:

- Quit Smoking: Smoking can exacerbate digestive problems and should be avoided.

- Limit Alcohol Intake: Alcohol can irritate the stomach lining and worsen symptoms. If you choose to drink, do so in moderation and avoid drinking on an empty stomach.

By adopting these eating habits and lifestyle changes, you can better manage your gastroparesis symptoms and improve your overall digestive health. The following chapters will provide more detailed guidance on incorporating these practices into your daily routine and offer practical tips for maintaining a healthy lifestyle with gastroparesis.

5. Managing Symptoms

Living with gastroparesis often means dealing with a range of challenging symptoms. Effective management of these symptoms is crucial for maintaining quality of life and overall health. This chapter focuses on strategies to manage common symptoms such as nausea and vomiting, bloating and gas, weight and nutrient absorption issues, and the use of medications and supplements.

Dealing with Nausea and Vomiting

Nausea and vomiting are among the most distressing symptoms of gastroparesis. These symptoms can severely impact daily activities and nutritional intake.

Strategies for Managing Nausea and Vomiting:

1. **Eat Small, Frequent Meals:** Smaller meals are less likely to trigger nausea. Avoid large meals that can cause the stomach to stretch and provoke symptoms.
2. **Avoid Trigger Foods:** High-fat and high-fiber foods can slow gastric emptying and increase nausea. Stick to low-fat, easily digestible options.
3. **Stay Hydrated:** Sipping clear fluids throughout the day can help manage nausea. Ginger tea, peppermint tea, and electrolyte solutions can be soothing.
4. **Medication:** Over-the-counter anti-nausea medications like ginger capsules or antihistamines (e.g., dimenhydrinate) can provide relief. Prescription medications such as ondansetron or prochlorperazine may be necessary in more severe cases.
5. **Acupressure and Acupuncture:** These alternative therapies have been shown to help

some individuals with nausea. Acupressure wristbands, for example, can be effective.

Strategies for Bloating and Gas

Bloating and gas are common complaints among those with gastroparesis, often leading to discomfort and embarrassment.

Tips for Reducing Bloating and Gas:

- 1. **Avoid Carbonated Beverages:** The bubbles in these drinks can introduce gas into your digestive system, leading to bloating.
- 2. **Eat Slowly and Chew Thoroughly:** Eating too quickly can cause you to swallow air, which contributes to gas and bloating. Thorough chewing aids in digestion.
- 3. **Choose Low-Fiber Foods:** High-fiber foods can ferment in the stomach and intestines, leading to gas. Opt for low-fiber alternatives.

- 4. **Gentle Exercise:** Light physical activity, such as walking, can help move gas through the digestive tract and reduce bloating.
- 5. **Over-the-Counter Remedies:** Simethicone-based products can help reduce gas. Herbal teas like peppermint or chamomile may also provide relief.

Managing Weight and Nutrient Absorption

Maintaining a healthy weight and ensuring proper nutrient absorption can be particularly challenging with gastroparesis. Malnutrition and weight loss are common concerns.

Tips for Managing Weight and Nutrient Absorption:

- 1. **Nutrient-Dense Foods:** Focus on foods that provide maximum nutrition in small portions. Smoothies with added protein powder, avocados, and nut butters (if tolerated) are good options.

- 2. **Liquid Nutrition:** Liquid meals, such as nutritional shakes, can be easier to tolerate and provide essential nutrients. Commercial products like Ensure or Boost can be beneficial.
- 3. **Frequent Small Meals:** Eating small, nutrient-dense meals throughout the day helps maintain calorie intake without overwhelming the digestive system.
- 4. **Work with a Dietitian:** A registered dietitian can help develop a personalized meal plan that meets your nutritional needs.
- 5. **Monitor Nutrient Levels:** Regular blood tests can help track levels of essential vitamins and minerals, ensuring deficiencies are identified and addressed promptly.

Medications and Supplements

Medications and supplements can play a vital role in managing gastroparesis symptoms.

However, it's essential to use them under the guidance of a healthcare professional.

Common Medications:

1. **Prokinetic Agents:** Medications like metoclopramide and erythromycin can stimulate stomach muscle contractions, helping to improve gastric emptying.
2. **Anti-Nausea Medications:** Drugs such as ondansetron and promethazine can help control nausea and vomiting.
3. **Pain Relief:** If abdominal pain is a significant issue, low-dose tricyclic antidepressants or gabapentin may be prescribed to manage discomfort.

Supplements:

1. **Multivitamins:** To address potential nutritional deficiencies, a daily multivitamin can be beneficial. Look for formulations specifically designed for individuals with digestive issues.

2. **Iron Supplements:** If blood tests reveal iron deficiency, iron supplements may be necessary. Liquid forms can be easier to tolerate.

3. **Vitamin B12:** Gastroparesis can interfere with B12 absorption. Sublingual or injectable forms of B12 may be required.

4. **Fiber Supplements:** If constipation is an issue, a soluble fiber supplement like psyllium can help. However, it should be used cautiously and under medical advice due to potential for increasing bloating and gas.

Using Medications and Supplements Safely:

- - **Follow Prescriptions:** Always take medications and supplements as prescribed by your healthcare provider.
- - **Monitor Side Effects:** Be aware of potential side effects and report any adverse reactions to your doctor.
- - **Avoid Self-Medicating:** Never start or stop a medication or supplement without consulting your healthcare provider.

By incorporating these strategies into your daily routine, you can better manage the symptoms of gastroparesis and improve your overall quality of life. The next chapter will provide a collection of gastroparesis-friendly recipes that are both nutritious and delicious, helping you to enjoy food while managing your condition effectively.

Part II:

Tips for Everyday Life

Managing gastroparesis effectively requires planning and adaptation, especially when navigating various everyday scenarios. This part offers practical advice on managing your condition while eating out, traveling, handling school and work lunches, and finding portable snacks and meals.

6. Managing Gastroparesis on the Go

Whether you're dining out, traveling, working, or at school, managing gastroparesis involves thoughtful preparation and strategic choices. Here's how to handle these situations effectively.

Eating Out and Social Situations

Eating out and participating in social events can be challenging with gastroparesis, but with a bit of planning, you can still enjoy these experiences.

Tips for Eating Out:

1. **Research and Plan Ahead:** Look at restaurant menus online before going out. Identify restaurants that offer simple, easily digestible options.
2. **Communicate Your Needs:** Inform the restaurant staff about your dietary restrictions. Request modifications to make dishes suitable for your condition.
3. **Choose Safe Options:** Opt for low-fat, low-fiber dishes like baked chicken, mashed potatoes, or well-cooked vegetables. Avoid rich sauces and fried foods.
4. **Ask for Small Portions:** Request smaller servings or share a meal to avoid overeating.

5. **Stay Hydrated:** Drink water or herbal teas, and avoid carbonated beverages that can cause bloating.

Handling Social Situations:

1. **Bring Your Own Food:** If you're unsure about the food options at a social event, consider bringing your own dish that meets your dietary needs.
2. **Focus on Beverages:** Choose beverages that are easy on your stomach, such as plain water or herbal teas.
3. **Participate in Activities:** Enjoy the social aspects of the event even if you're not eating. Engaging in conversation and activities can make the event enjoyable.

Traveling with Gastroparesis

Traveling can present additional challenges, but with careful planning, you can manage your condition effectively.

Travel Tips:

1. **Prepare and Pack:** Pack non-perishable snacks that adhere to your dietary needs, such as low-fat crackers, applesauce, or protein bars.
2. **Plan Meals in Advance:** Research dining options at your destination and locate places that offer suitable food.
3. **Stay Hydrated:** Carry a refillable water bottle and ensure you have access to clean drinking water.
4. **Stick to a Routine:** Maintain your eating schedule as closely as possible, even while traveling.
5. **Carry Medications:** Bring all necessary medications and supplements, and keep them in their original containers for security checks.

Traveling by Air:

1. **Inform Airline Staff:** Notify the airline about your dietary needs. Request special meal options if available.

2. Carry Medications and Documentation:

Keep medications in your carry-on, and bring any required documentation, such as a doctor's note, if needed.

School and Work Lunches

Managing gastroparesis during school or work requires preparation and organization to ensure you have suitable meal options.

Tips for School and Work Lunches:

1. **Prepare Meals in Advance:** Plan and pack your meals the night before. Use insulated containers to keep food fresh.

2. **Choose Portable Options:** Opt for meals that are easy to transport and eat, such as small sandwiches made with soft bread or easy-to-digest salads.

3. **Communicate Your Needs:** Inform your school or workplace about your dietary restrictions. Request access to a refrigerator or microwave if needed.

4. **Pack Extra Snacks:** Keep additional snacks on hand in case you get hungry between meals or if your meal schedule changes.

Ideas for School and Work Lunches:

1. **Soft Wraps:** Fill soft wraps with lean proteins and easily digestible vegetables.
2. **Mini Quiches:** Prepare mini quiches with low-fat ingredients for a portable and nutritious option.
3. **Smoothies:** Blend fruits, yogurt, and protein powder into a smoothie that is easy to consume and digest.

Portable Snacks and Meals

Having portable snacks and meals ready can help you manage gastroparesis while on the go, ensuring you stay nourished without disrupting your routine.

Ideas for Portable Snacks:

1. **Low-Fat Crackers:** Easy to pack and digest, these can be paired with low-fat cheese or spreads.

2. **Applesauce Cups:** Convenient and gentle on the stomach.

3. **Protein Bars:** Choose bars that are low in fat and fiber.

4. **Smoothie Packs:** Pre-made or homemade smoothie packs are portable and easy to consume. Use resealable bags or containers.

Ideas for Portable Meals:

1. **Soup in a Thermos:** Prepare and pack a gentle soup in an insulated thermos to keep it warm and easy to consume.

2. **Mini Sandwiches:** Use soft bread and fillings like lean meats or light spreads for a manageable meal.

3. **Cooked Pasta:** Small portions of well-cooked pasta with mild sauces are easy to digest and transport.

By following these tips, you can better navigate daily life with gastroparesis, making it easier to manage your condition while enjoying a variety of activities and responsibilities. The subsequent chapters will offer further guidance on integrating these practices into your lifestyle and provide additional recipes tailored to your dietary needs.

7. Emotional and Mental Well-being

Living with gastroparesis can take a toll on your emotional and mental health. Managing a chronic illness involves more than just addressing physical symptoms—it's also crucial to take care of your emotional well-being. This chapter focuses on strategies for coping with chronic illness, managing stress, building support networks, and incorporating mindfulness and relaxation practices into your daily life.

Coping with Chronic Illness

Dealing with a chronic condition like gastroparesis can be overwhelming and affect your overall sense of well-being. Here are some strategies to help you cope:

1. **Acknowledge Your Feelings:** It's normal to experience a range of emotions, including frustration, sadness, or anxiety. Recognizing and accepting these feelings is the first step in managing them.

2. **Set Realistic Goals:** Focus on what you can control and set achievable goals. This could include managing symptoms, adjusting to new routines, or making small lifestyle changes.

3. **Seek Professional Help:** Consider speaking with a mental health professional, such as a therapist or counselor, who can help you navigate the emotional challenges of living with a chronic illness.

4. **Stay Informed:** Educate yourself about gastroparesis and its management.

Understanding your condition can help you feel more in control and reduce anxiety about the unknown.

5. **Practice Self-Compassion:** Be kind to yourself. Recognize that managing a chronic illness is challenging, and it's okay to have difficult days.

Stress Management Techniques

Chronic stress can exacerbate symptoms and negatively impact your health. Effective stress management is essential for maintaining your emotional and physical well-being.

1. **Deep Breathing Exercises:** Practice deep breathing to help calm your mind and reduce stress. Try inhaling deeply through your nose, holding for a few seconds, and exhaling slowly through your mouth.

2. **Progressive Muscle Relaxation:** This technique involves tensing and then relaxing

different muscle groups in your body. It can help release physical tension and promote relaxation.

3. **Regular Exercise:** Engage in light physical activities such as walking or stretching. Exercise can help reduce stress, improve mood, and boost overall well-being.

4. **Time Management:** Organize your daily tasks and prioritize activities to reduce feelings of being overwhelmed. Break larger tasks into smaller, manageable steps.

5. **Engage in Hobbies:** Spend time on activities that you enjoy and that bring you satisfaction, whether it's reading, gardening, or crafting.

Support Networks and Resources

Building a support network and accessing resources can provide emotional support and practical help in managing your condition.

1. **Connect with Support Groups:** Join local or online support groups for people with gastroparesis. Sharing experiences and advice with others who understand your situation can be comforting.

2. **Communicate with Family and Friends:** Keep open lines of communication with those close to you. Share your needs and concerns so they can offer support and understanding.

3. **Seek Professional Support:** Consider working with a social worker or patient advocate who can help you navigate healthcare systems, manage insurance issues, and find additional resources.

4. **Utilize Educational Resources:** Access educational materials and resources from reputable organizations like the Gastroparesis Patient Association or the National Institute of Diabetes and Digestive and Kidney Diseases (NIDDK).

5. **Involve Your Healthcare Team:** Regularly discuss your emotional and mental health with your healthcare providers. They can offer guidance, recommend resources, and adjust your treatment plan as needed.

Mindfulness and Relaxation Practices

Incorporating mindfulness and relaxation practices into your daily routine can help manage stress, improve emotional resilience, and enhance your overall quality of life.

1. **Mindfulness Meditation:** Practice mindfulness meditation to stay present and focused. Simple techniques include paying attention to your breath, observing your thoughts without judgment, and grounding yourself in the present moment.

2. **Guided Imagery:** Use guided imagery to visualize calming and positive scenarios. This technique can help reduce stress and create a sense of relaxation.

3. **Yoga and Stretching:** Gentle yoga and stretching exercises can promote relaxation, improve flexibility, and help with stress management. Look for classes or online resources specifically tailored to individuals with chronic conditions.

4. **Journaling:** Keep a journal to express your thoughts and feelings. Writing about your experiences can help process emotions and provide insights into your emotional state.

5. **Relaxation Techniques:** Incorporate relaxation techniques such as listening to calming music, taking warm baths, or practicing aromatherapy with essential oils.

By focusing on emotional and mental well-being, you can better manage the challenges of living with gastroparesis and enhance your overall quality of life. The next chapters will provide further guidance on practical tips and strategies for integrating these practices into your daily routine.

Part III:

Recipes to Manage Digestive Health

Eating well is crucial for managing gastroparesis. In this section, you'll find recipes tailored to be gentle on the digestive system while providing essential nutrients. These breakfast options are designed to be easy to digest and satisfying.

8. Breakfasts

1. Easy-to-Digest Smoothies

Smoothies are an excellent option for breakfast as they can be tailored to be gentle on the stomach while still providing necessary nutrients.

Recipe: Banana and Almond Smoothie

Ingredients:
- 1 ripe banana
- 1 cup almond milk (unsweetened)
- 1 tablespoon almond butter
- 1 teaspoon honey (optional)
- 1/4 teaspoon vanilla extract

Instructions:
1. Peel and slice the banana.
2. In a blender, combine the banana, almond milk, almond butter, honey, and vanilla extract.
3. Blend until smooth.
4. Pour into a glass and serve immediately.

2. Soft and Nourishing Breakfast Bowls

Breakfast bowls are versatile and can be made with ingredients that are easy on the digestive system. They are soft and easy to digest, making them suitable for those with gastroparesis.

Recipe: Creamy Oatmeal Bowl

Ingredients:
- 1/2 cup rolled oats
- 1 cup water or low-fat milk
- 1/4 cup applesauce (unsweetened)
- 1/2 teaspoon cinnamon
- 1/2 banana, sliced

Instructions:
1. In a saucepan, combine oats and water or milk. Bring to a boil.
2. Reduce heat and simmer, stirring occasionally, until oats are tender (about 5 minutes).
3. Stir in applesauce and cinnamon.
4. Serve topped with sliced banana.

3. Light and Fluffy Pancakes

Pancakes can be made gentle on the stomach by using easy-to-digest ingredients. These light and fluffy pancakes are designed to be well-tolerated.

Recipe: Light Pancakes

Ingredients:

- 1 cup all-purpose flour
- 1 tablespoon sugar
- 1 teaspoon baking powder
- 1/2 teaspoon salt
- 1 cup low-fat milk
- 1 large egg
- 1 tablespoon vegetable oil

Instructions:

1. In a bowl, whisk together flour, sugar, baking powder, and salt.
2. In another bowl, mix milk, egg, and vegetable oil.
3. Combine wet and dry ingredients, stirring until just blended.
4. Heat a non-stick skillet over medium heat and lightly grease with cooking spray or a small amount of oil.
5. Pour batter onto the skillet, using about 1/4 cup for each pancake. Cook until bubbles form on the surface, then flip and cook until golden brown.

6. Serve warm, topped with a small amount of maple syrup or fruit puree if desired.

These breakfast recipes are designed to provide a nutritious start to your day while being mindful of the dietary needs associated with gastroparesis. The next section will offer more recipes and ideas for other meals throughout the day.

9. Lunches

Lunches for those managing gastroparesis should be gentle on the digestive system while providing necessary nutrients. Here are some easy-to-digest and satisfying options for lunch.

Simple and Satisfying Soups

Soups can be a comforting and easily digestible lunch option. They are often gentle on the stomach and can be packed with nutrients.

Recipe: Creamy Chicken and Rice Soup

Ingredients:
- 1 cup cooked, shredded chicken breast
- 1/2 cup cooked white rice
- 2 cups low-sodium chicken broth
- 1/2 cup carrots, finely diced
- 1/4 cup celery, finely diced
- 1/2 cup low-fat milk
- 1 tablespoon olive oil
- Salt and pepper to taste

Instructions:
1. In a large pot, heat olive oil over medium heat. Add carrots and celery, and cook until softened (about 5 minutes).
2. Add chicken broth and bring to a boil.
3. Reduce heat and simmer for 10 minutes.
4. Stir in cooked chicken and rice.
5. Gradually add milk, stirring continuously.
6. Season with salt and pepper to taste. Heat through but do not boil.
7. Serve warm.

Light Salads with Digestive-Friendly Dressings

Salads can be tailored to be gentle on the digestive system by using soft ingredients and mild dressings.

Recipe: Soft Spinach Salad with Yogurt Dressing

Ingredients:
- 2 cups baby spinach
- 1/4 cup finely shredded carrots
- 1/4 cup cooked and cooled quinoa
- 1/4 cup plain Greek yogurt
- 1 tablespoon lemon juice
- 1 teaspoon honey
- Salt to taste

Instructions:
1. In a large bowl, combine spinach, shredded carrots, and quinoa.
2. In a small bowl, mix Greek yogurt, lemon juice, honey, and salt until well combined.

3. Drizzle the yogurt dressing over the salad and toss gently.

4. Serve immediately or chill until ready to eat.

Soft Sandwiches and Wraps

Sandwiches and wraps can be made easy to digest by using soft ingredients and avoiding high-fiber fillings.

Recipe: Turkey and Avocado Soft Wrap

Ingredients:
- 1 soft whole wheat or white tortilla
- 2-3 slices of lean turkey breast
- 1/4 avocado, sliced
- 1/4 cup low-fat cream cheese
- 1/4 cup baby spinach (optional)

Instructions:
1. Spread cream cheese evenly over the tortilla.
2. Layer turkey slices and avocado on top.
3. Add baby spinach if desired.
4. Roll the tortilla tightly and slice in half.

5. Serve immediately or wrap tightly for an on-the-go meal.

These lunch recipes are designed to be gentle on the stomach while providing nourishment and variety. The following section will include more dinner recipes and ideas to complement these meal options.

10. Dinners

Dinner should be comforting and easy to digest, providing a satisfying end to your day. Here are some dinner ideas that are gentle on the stomach and suitable for those managing gastroparesis.

Gentle-on-the-Stomach Casseroles

Casseroles can be a convenient and nutritious option for dinner. Opt for recipes that use easily digestible ingredients and avoid heavy or fatty components.

Recipe: Chicken and Rice Casserole

Ingredients:
- 2 cups cooked, shredded chicken breast
- 1 cup cooked white rice
- 1 cup low-sodium chicken broth
- 1/2 cup low-fat cream of chicken soup
- 1/2 cup peas (cooked and soft)
- 1/2 cup shredded low-fat cheese
- 1/4 teaspoon dried thyme
- Salt and pepper to taste

Instructions:
1. Preheat oven to 350°F (175°C).
2. In a large bowl, combine chicken, rice, chicken broth, cream of chicken soup, peas, and half of the cheese. Mix well.
3. Transfer mixture to a baking dish and top with remaining cheese.
4. Bake for 20-25 minutes, or until the casserole is heated through and the cheese is melted and bubbly.
5. Let cool slightly before serving.

Tender Protein Dishes

Protein dishes can be made tender and easy to digest by cooking them slowly or using tender cuts of meat.

Recipe: Baked Lemon Herb Salmon

Ingredients:
- 4 salmon fillets
- 2 tablespoons olive oil
- 1 tablespoon lemon juice
- 1 teaspoon dried dill
- 1 teaspoon dried parsley
- Salt and pepper to taste

Instructions:
1. Preheat oven to 375°F (190°C).
2. Place salmon fillets on a baking sheet lined with parchment paper.
3. In a small bowl, mix olive oil, lemon juice, dill, parsley, salt, and pepper.
4. Brush the mixture over the salmon fillets.

5. Bake for 15-20 minutes, or until the salmon is cooked through and flakes easily with a fork.
6. Serve with a side of rice or soft vegetables.

Easy-to-Digest Vegetables and Sides

Side dishes can complement your main course and should be prepared to be gentle on the stomach.

Recipe: Steamed Carrots and Potatoes

Ingredients:
- 2 medium potatoes, peeled and diced
- 2 cups baby carrots
- 1 tablespoon olive oil
- Salt to taste

Instructions:
1. Steam potatoes and carrots until tender (about 10-15 minutes).
2. Transfer to a bowl and toss with olive oil and salt.
3. Serve warm as a side dish.

Recipe: Mashed Sweet Potatoes

Ingredients:
- 2 large sweet potatoes, peeled and cubed
- 1/4 cup low-fat milk
- 1 tablespoon butter or margarine
- Salt and a pinch of cinnamon (optional)

Instructions:
1. Boil sweet potatoes in a pot of water until tender (about 15-20 minutes).
2. Drain and return to the pot.
3. Add milk, butter, and a pinch of cinnamon if desired. Mash until smooth.
4. Season with salt to taste and serve warm.

These dinner recipes are designed to be soothing and easy to digest, ensuring you enjoy a nourishing and satisfying meal. The next section will continue with more meal ideas and recipes to help manage your gastroparesis effectively.

11. Snacks and Small Meals

Snacks and small meals are essential for maintaining energy levels and managing gastroparesis. The following recipes focus on gentle, nutritious options that are easy on the digestive system.

Nutritious Smoothie Recipes

Smoothies can be a great way to get vitamins and minerals while being gentle on the stomach. Here are some simple and nutritious smoothie recipes:

Recipe: Banana and Spinach Smoothie

Ingredients:
- 1 ripe banana
- 1 cup fresh spinach leaves
- 1/2 cup plain Greek yogurt
- 1/2 cup almond milk (or any low-fat milk)
- 1 tablespoon honey (optional)

Instructions:

1. Peel and slice the banana.
2. In a blender, combine the banana, spinach, Greek yogurt, and almond milk.
3. Blend until smooth.
4. Add honey if desired for extra sweetness.
5. Serve immediately.

Recipe: Peach and Oat Smoothie

Ingredients:
- 1 cup frozen peaches
- 1/2 cup rolled oats
- 1 cup low-fat milk or almond milk
- 1/2 teaspoon vanilla extract

Instructions:

1. In a blender, combine frozen peaches, oats, milk, and vanilla extract.
2. Blend until smooth.
3. Serve immediately.

Digestive-Friendly Snack Bars

Snack bars can be a convenient way to manage hunger and get nutrients. These recipes focus on ingredients that are gentle on the digestive system.

Recipe: Almond and Date Energy Bars

Ingredients:
- 1 cup almonds
- 1 cup pitted dates
- 1/2 cup unsweetened shredded coconut
- 1 tablespoon chia seeds (optional)

Instructions:
1. In a food processor, blend almonds and dates until finely chopped and combined.
2. Add shredded coconut and chia seeds if using. Pulse until mixed.
3. Press the mixture firmly into a lined 8x8-inch baking dish.
4. Refrigerate for at least 1 hour before cutting into bars.

Recipe: Rice Cake and Nut Butter Bars

Ingredients:
- 2 cups rice cakes, crushed
- 1/2 cup almond or peanut butter
- 1/4 cup honey
- 1/4 cup dried cranberries (optional)

Instructions:
1. In a large bowl, combine crushed rice cakes, nut butter, and honey.
2. Mix until well combined. Stir in dried cranberries if using.
3. Press the mixture into a lined baking dish.
4. Refrigerate for at least 1 hour before cutting into bars.

Soft and Easy-to-Eat Snacks

Soft snacks are ideal for those managing gastroparesis, as they are gentle on the stomach and easy to digest.

Recipe: Mashed Avocado on Soft Toast

Ingredients:
- 1 ripe avocado
- 1 slice of soft, white or whole wheat bread
- A squeeze of lemon juice
- Salt to taste

Instructions:
1. Toast the bread lightly, if desired.
2. Mash the avocado in a bowl and add a squeeze of lemon juice and salt.
3. Spread the mashed avocado on the soft toast.
4. Serve immediately.

Recipe: Greek Yogurt with Honey and Soft Fruit

Ingredients:
- 1/2 cup plain Greek yogurt
- 1 tablespoon honey
- 1/4 cup soft fruit, such as ripe bananas or peeled apples

Instructions:
1. Spoon Greek yogurt into a bowl.

2. Drizzle with honey.

3. Top with soft fruit and serve.

Recipe: Applesauce with Cinnamon

Ingredients:
- 1 cup unsweetened applesauce
- 1/2 teaspoon ground cinnamon

Instructions:
1. Stir cinnamon into applesauce.
2. Serve chilled or at room temperature.

These recipes offer gentle, nutritious options for snacks and small meals, helping to manage symptoms and support overall well-being. The next section will cover additional meal ideas and recipes to round out your diet.

12. Desserts

Desserts can be a delightful part of a meal, even when managing gastroparesis. These recipes are designed to be gentle on the stomach while providing a satisfying end to your meal.

Light and Fluffy Cakes

Light cakes can be a treat that's easy on the digestive system. Opt for recipes that use simple, easily digestible ingredients.

Recipe: Vanilla Angel Food Cake

Ingredients:
- 1 cup egg whites (about 8 large eggs)
- 1 cup granulated sugar
- 1 cup cake flour
- 1 teaspoon vanilla extract
- 1/4 teaspoon cream of tartar

Instructions:
1. Preheat oven to 350°F (175°C). Have an ungreased angel food cake pan ready.
2. In a mixing bowl, beat egg whites and cream of tartar until soft peaks form.

3. Gradually add sugar, beating until stiff peaks form.
4. Gently fold in cake flour and vanilla extract.
5. Pour batter into the pan and smooth the top.
6. Bake for 35-40 minutes, or until the cake springs back when touched.
7. Cool upside down before removing from the pan.

Recipe: Lemon Sponge Cake

Ingredients:
- 1 cup cake flour
- 1/2 cup granulated sugar
- 1/4 cup lemon juice
- 1/4 cup vegetable oil
- 3 large eggs
- 1 teaspoon baking powder

Instructions:
1. Preheat oven to 350°F (175°C). Grease and flour an 8-inch round cake pan.
2. In a bowl, whisk together flour, sugar, and baking powder.

3. In another bowl, beat eggs, then add lemon juice and vegetable oil.

4. Combine wet and dry ingredients, mixing until just blended.

5. Pour batter into the prepared pan.

6. Bake for 25-30 minutes, or until a toothpick inserted into the center comes out clean.

7. Cool before serving.

Soft and Creamy Puddings

Puddings are a soothing dessert that can be made with easy-to-digest ingredients.

Recipe: Vanilla Custard Pudding

Ingredients:
- 2 cups low-fat milk
- 1/4 cup granulated sugar
- 2 tablespoons cornstarch
- 1/2 teaspoon vanilla extract
- A pinch of salt

Instructions:

1. In a saucepan, whisk together milk, sugar, cornstarch, and salt.
2. Cook over medium heat, stirring constantly until the mixture thickens and begins to bubble.
3. Remove from heat and stir in vanilla extract.
4. Pour into individual serving dishes and let cool.
5. Chill in the refrigerator before serving.

Recipe: Chocolate Avocado Pudding

Ingredients:
- 1 ripe avocado
- 1/4 cup unsweetened cocoa powder
- 1/4 cup honey or maple syrup
- 1/4 cup almond milk (or any low-fat milk)
- 1/2 teaspoon vanilla extract

Instructions:
1. In a blender, combine avocado, cocoa powder, honey, almond milk, and vanilla extract.
2. Blend until smooth and creamy.
3. Spoon into serving dishes and refrigerate for at least 30 minutes before serving.

Digestive-Friendly Frozen Treats

Frozen treats can be a refreshing and gentle way to enjoy dessert. These recipes are designed to be easy on the stomach.

Recipe: Frozen Banana Bites

Ingredients:
- 2 ripe bananas
- 1/4 cup almond butter or peanut butter
- 1/4 cup dark chocolate chips (optional)

Instructions:
1. Slice bananas into bite-sized pieces.
2. Spread a small amount of almond butter on one side of each banana slice.
3. Optional: Melt dark chocolate chips and dip each banana slice in the chocolate.
4. Place banana slices on a baking sheet lined with parchment paper.
5. Freeze until solid, then store in a container in the freezer.

Recipe: Mango Coconut Sorbet

Ingredients:
- 2 cups frozen mango chunks
- 1/2 cup coconut milk
- 2 tablespoons honey or maple syrup

Instructions:
1. In a blender or food processor, combine frozen mango, coconut milk, and honey.
2. Blend until smooth.
3. Pour mixture into a freezer-safe container and freeze for at least 2 hours.
4. Scoop and serve.

These dessert recipes offer gentle, delicious options that fit within a gastroparesis-friendly diet, providing a sweet end to your meals while being easy on your digestive system.

13. Beverages

Choosing the right beverages is crucial for maintaining hydration and nourishment, especially when managing gastroparesis. Here are some gentle and beneficial drink options:

Hydrating and Nourishing Drinks

These drinks are designed to keep you hydrated and provide essential nutrients without irritating the digestive system.

Recipe: Cucumber-Melon Refresher

Ingredients:
- 1 cup cucumber, peeled and sliced
- 1 cup honeydew melon, cubed
- 1 cup water or coconut water
- A few mint leaves (optional)

Instructions:
1. Blend cucumber and honeydew melon with water or coconut water until smooth.
2. Strain through a fine mesh sieve if desired for a smoother texture.

3. Garnish with mint leaves if using and serve chilled.

Recipe: Aloe Vera Juice

Ingredients:
- 1 cup aloe vera juice (unsweetened)
- 1/2 cup apple juice
- 1 teaspoon lemon juice

Instructions:
1. Combine aloe vera juice, apple juice, and lemon juice in a glass.
2. Stir well and serve chilled.

Herbal Teas and Infusions

Herbal teas and infusions can be soothing and are often easy on the stomach. They provide comfort and can aid digestion.

Recipe: Peppermint Tea

Ingredients:

- 1 peppermint tea bag or 1/4 cup fresh peppermint leaves
- 1 cup hot water
- 1 teaspoon honey (optional)

Instructions:

1. Steep the tea bag or peppermint leaves in hot water for 5-7 minutes.
2. Remove the tea bag or strain out the leaves.
3. Add honey if desired and serve warm.

Recipe: Ginger-Lemon Tea

Ingredients:
- 1-inch piece of fresh ginger, sliced
- 1 cup hot water
- Juice of 1/2 lemon
- 1 teaspoon honey (optional)

Instructions:

1. Boil ginger slices in hot water for 5-10 minutes.
2. Strain the ginger out and stir in lemon juice and honey if using.

3. Serve warm.

Smoothies and Shakes

Smoothies and shakes are versatile and can be tailored to be gentle on the stomach while providing essential nutrients.

Recipe: Creamy Banana Smoothie

Ingredients:
- 1 ripe banana
- 1/2 cup plain Greek yogurt
- 1/2 cup low-fat milk or almond milk
- 1 tablespoon honey (optional)

Instructions:
1. Blend banana, Greek yogurt, and milk until smooth.
2. Add honey for sweetness if desired.
3. Serve immediately.

Recipe: Berry Almond Shake

Ingredients:
- 1/2 cup frozen mixed berries
- 1 cup almond milk
- 1 tablespoon almond butter
- 1/2 teaspoon vanilla extract

Instructions:
1. Blend berries, almond milk, almond butter, and vanilla extract until smooth.
2. Serve immediately.

These beverage options are designed to be soothing and nourishing, making them suitable for those managing gastroparesis. They offer a variety of flavors and benefits while being gentle on the digestive system.

Conclusion

14. Living Well with Gastroparesis

Living well with gastroparesis involves a comprehensive approach that includes understanding the condition, implementing effective management strategies, and staying informed about new developments. Here's a summary of how to navigate this journey:

Recap of Key Points

1. **Understanding Gastroparesis:** Gastroparesis is a disorder affecting stomach emptying. Key symptoms include nausea, vomiting, and abdominal bloating. Understanding its impact on daily life helps in managing the condition effectively.

2. **Dietary Guidelines:** A diet tailored to gastroparesis involves small, frequent meals that are low in fiber and fat. Focusing on

well-cooked, soft foods can reduce symptoms and improve nutrient absorption.

3. **Meal Planning and Preparation:** Careful planning and preparation of meals can help manage symptoms and ensure a balanced diet. Emphasizing foods that are easy to digest while maintaining nutritional value is crucial.

4. **Eating Habits and Lifestyle Changes:** Adopting specific eating habits, such as eating slowly and staying hydrated, along with lifestyle changes like stress management and regular physical activity, can enhance digestion and overall well-being.

5. **Managing Symptoms:** Effective management includes addressing nausea, bloating, and other symptoms with appropriate strategies and medications. Working closely with healthcare professionals to tailor treatment is important.

6. **Everyday Life Adjustments:** Practical adjustments in daily life, including when eating

out or traveling, help maintain a comfortable routine. Carrying gastroparesis-friendly snacks and planning ahead can make a significant difference.

7. **Emotional and Mental Well-being:** Coping with a chronic illness requires attention to mental health. Engaging in stress-reducing activities, seeking support, and practicing mindfulness can support emotional resilience.

8. **Recipes and Meal Ideas:** Enjoying a variety of recipes that adhere to dietary guidelines can make meals more enjoyable. From breakfasts to desserts, choosing recipes that are gentle on the stomach can improve quality of life.

Ongoing Management and Monitoring

1. **Regular Check-ups:** Routine visits to healthcare providers are essential for monitoring the condition, adjusting treatments, and addressing any emerging issues.

2. **Symptom Tracking:** Keeping a record of food intake and symptoms helps identify patterns and triggers, allowing for more personalized management strategies.

3. **Nutritional Assessment:** Regular assessments by a dietitian ensure nutritional needs are met and any deficiencies are addressed.

4. **Treatment Adjustments:** Being open to adjustments in treatment plans based on symptom changes or new medical insights helps manage the condition more effectively.

Staying Informed and Up-to-Date

1. **Continuous Education:** Staying informed about gastroparesis through reliable sources and professional advice helps in adapting to new information and treatments.

2. **Support Networks:** Connecting with support groups and communities provides emotional

support and practical advice from others with similar experiences.

3. **Resource Utilization:** Utilizing educational materials, symptom-tracking tools, and meal-planning resources can enhance daily management and improve overall quality of life.

By integrating these strategies, individuals with gastroparesis can effectively manage their condition and lead a fulfilling life.

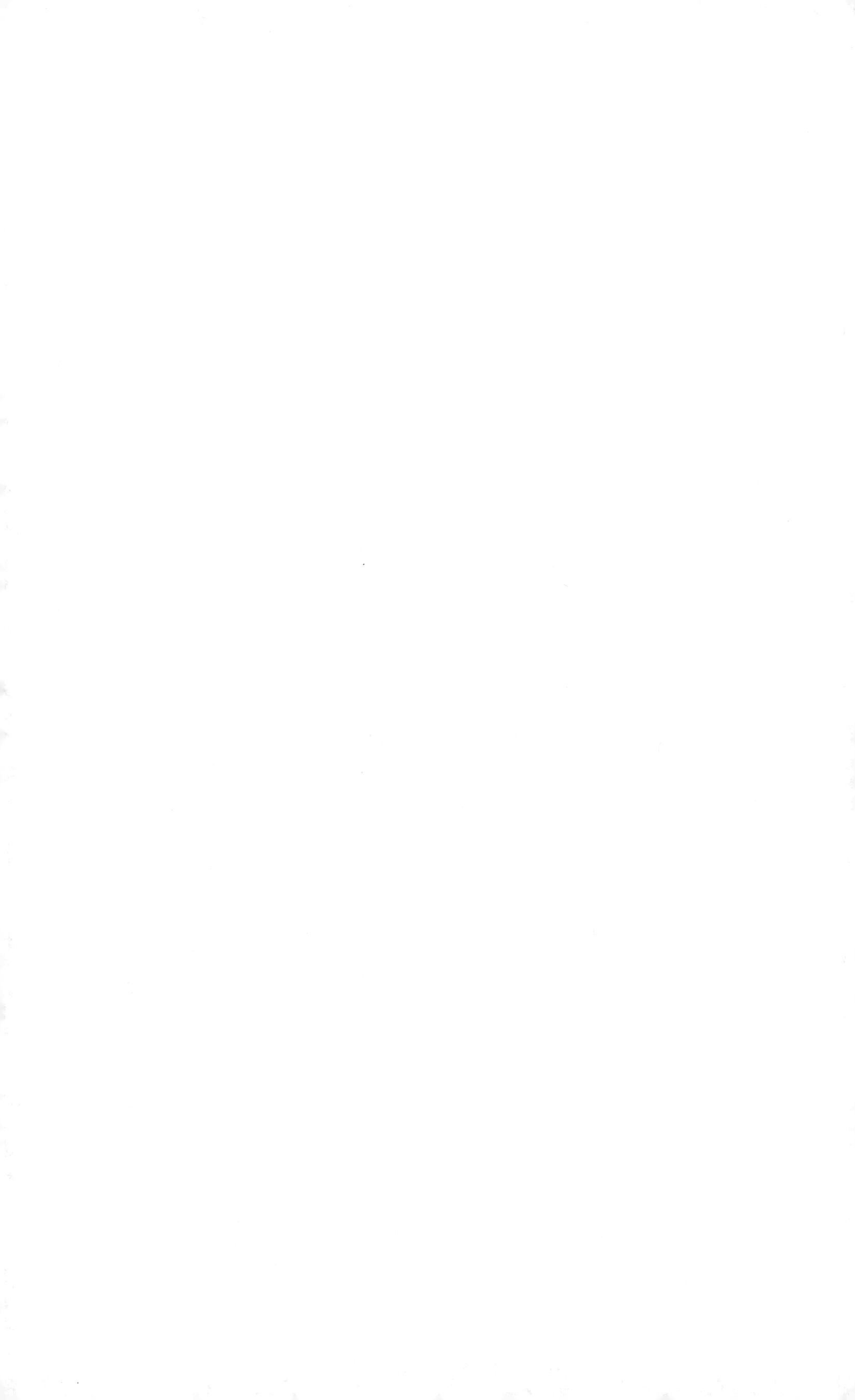